Starter Vegetable Gardens

The Complete guide step by step

Author

Laura J. Hahne

Contents

You may wonder why I'm planting a garden. The sweet, juicy flavors and vibrant textures will astound you if you've never tried garden-fresh vegetables before (which many people haven't!). Nothing like fresh vegetables, particularly if you can raise them yourself.

CHOOSE THE BEST LOCATION FOR YOUR BUSINESS

It's critical to choose the right spot for your garden. A bad site might lead to bad produce! Here are some pointers on how to pick a good web page:

1. Choose a sunny spot to grow your plants. The majority of vegetables require at least 6 hours of direct sunlight each day to thrive. A few vegetables can be grown in partial shade.

2. Make sure the soil is moist and well-drained. Plant vegetables in a raised bed if your soil is badly drained (water pools). Till the soil and remove the rocks if it is rocky.

3. Grow your plants in a secure setting. Avoid placing your young plants in areas where strong winds may knock them over or prevent pollinators from doing their job. or do you want to plant in an area with a lot of foot traffic or is prone to flooding? Plant where Goldilocks would be pleased.

2

START SMALL WHEN CREATING A PLOT!

Remember, it's preferable to be proud of a small garden than to be frustrated by a large one!

One of the most common rookie mistakes is planning too much too soon—way more than anyone could possibly eat or desire! If you don't want zucchini in your attic, plan your garden carefully. Start small and grow only what you're sure you'll eat.

Here are some ideas for a good-sized beginner vegetable garden that can feed a family of four for a summer, with some extra for canning and freezing (or giving away to jealo us neighbors).

1. Make your garden 11 rows wide by 80 feet long.

3

To maximize the sun's exposure, the rows should run north and south.

2. Make sure you have access to your plants so you can weed and harvest them. The general rule is that no more than four feet of plants should be allowed to grow without being accessible. Make sure you can easily reach the row or bed's center.

(Note: If this garden is too big for your needs, you can skip the 11th row or make the rows shorter.)

VEGETABLE SELECTION

Here are some pointers on how to select vegetables:

1. Decide on your favorite foods (and those of your family). If no one enjoys the number four,

Don't bother planting Brussels sprouts!

2. Consider how many vegetables your family will consume. Make sure you're not overplanting. (Of course, you could always give your vegetables to someone who needs them.)

3. Think about what vegetables are available at your local supermarket. Instead of the cabbage or carrots that are available, you might want to grow tomatillo. Garden lettuce and tomatoes, for example, are so much better when grown at home that it's almost a shame not to consider them. Herbs grown at home are also significantly less expensive than herbs purchased at a grocery store.

4. Is it possible to take a vacation during the summer? In the middle of summer, tomatoes and zucchinis are ready to harvest. If you're going to be gone for a portion of the summer, you'll need someone to look after the d rops or they'll suffer. Planting cool-season crops like lettuce and kale, as well as root vegetables, is another option.

5. Make use of high-quality materials, as indicated by the ds. Although seed packets are less costly than individual plants, your money and time are wasted if the seeds do not germinate. Spending a few extra cents on seeds in the spring for the following year's

harvest will result in higher yields. Purchasing seeds directly from the nursery is less expensive and of higher quality if you plan ahead of time.

5

WHAT SHOULD I PLANT AND WHEN SHOULD I PLANT IT?

This process is simple if you only want to grow two or three tornato plants. However, if you want to grow a complete garden, you must consider the following factors:

What will be the fate of each vegetable?

When do you need to plant each vegetable?

Here are some suggestions for how to arrange your vegetables:

1. There are "cool-season" vegetables that grow in the spring (e.g., lettuce, spinach, root vegetables) and "warm-season" vegetables that don't grow until the soil warms up (eq,

tomatoes, peppers). Plant cool-season crops after the first frost of the season, and then warm-season crops later in the season in the same area.

2. Grow tali vegetables in your garden (such as pole beans or a trellis or sweet com)

6

so that they don't shade the shorter plants on the north side of the garden Save a section of your garden for small cool-season vegetables if you do get some shade. If shade is unavoidable in some areas of your garden, use those spots to grow cool-season vegetables that benefit from the shade as the weather warms.

3. Annual vegetables make up the majority of the vegetable garden (planted each year). Provide permanent locarions or beds if you plan to grow "perennial" crops like asparagus, rhubarb, or herbs.

4. Take into account the fact that some crops mature quickly and have a short harvest season (radjshes, bush beans). Plants with a longer rime period, such as tomatoes, are more common. On the seed packet, you'll find "days to maturity." Beans, beets, carrots, cabbage, kohlrabi, lettuce, rarushes, rutabagas, spinach, and turnips are examples of vegetables that produce multiple crops per season.

Planrings should be spaced out. You don't want to plant your lettuce seeds or harvest your lettuce at the same time! Planrings should be spaced out by a few weeks to keep things fresh.

When is the best time to plant?

Every region has its own planning rime based on its weather, and each vegetable table has its own temperature preferences. See\s7

The Almanac's Best Planting Dates is a gardening calendar that is tailored to your region's frost dates. Simply type in your zip code to get started.

See our individua for detailed planting instructions. Over 100 popular vegetables, herbs, and fruits are covered in these grow guides. We give detailed instructions for planting, growing, and harvesting each crop, including watering, fertilizing, and pest control!!

Special benefits come with organic vegetable gardens.

It is both fun and rewarding to grow your own vegetables. You only need some good soil and a few plants to get started, Ali. But, in order to be a truly successful vegetable gardener - and to do so organically - you'll need to know how to keep your plants healthy and vigorous. The fundamentals are as follows:

For organic gardeners, "feed the soil" has become a mantra, and for good reason. Crop plants are, in fact, "fed" directly with synthetic fertilizers in conventional chemical agriculture.

This type of chemical force-feeding, when taken to extremes, can gradually degrade the soil. And turn it from a nutrient-rich environment teeming with microorganisms, insects, and other life forms into an inert growing medium that serves primarily to anchor the roots of the plants while providing little or no nutrition in and of itself.

While various fertilizers and mineral nutrients (agricultural lime, rock phosphate, greensand, and so on) should be added to the organic garden on a regular basis, organic matter is by far the most useful substance for building and maintaining a healthy, well-balanced soil.

There are a variety of ways to incorporate organic matter into your soil, including 9

Compost, shredded leaves, animal manure, or cover crops are examples of materials that can be used.

Organic matter improves soil fertility, structure, and tilth. Organic matter, in particular, provides a steady supply of nitrogen and other nutrients that plants require to thrive. It's also a good source of food for soil microbes. These nutrients become available to plants as soil organisms carry out the processes of decay and decomposition. Read Building Healthy Soil for more information.

Use Space Wisely

Your garden's location (the amount of sunlight it receives, its proximity to a source of water, and its protection from frost and wind) is critical. Making the most of your garden space is equally important when growing vegetables.

Many people fantasize about having a large vegetable table garden, a sprawling plot of land large enough to grow anything they want, including space-hungry crops like corn, dried beans, pumpkins and winter squash, as well as melons, cucumbers, and watermelons. Go for it if you have the space and, more importantly, the time and energy to maintain a large garden. However, whether I O or not, vegetable gardens that make efficient use of growing space are much easier to maintain.

It could be a couple of containers on the patio or a 50-by-100-foot plot in the backyard. For beginners, raised beds are a good option because they make the garden easier to manage.

Getting Rid of Your Rows is a must-do task for anyone who wants to

Converting from traditional row planting to 3- or 4-foot-wide raised beds is the first way to maximize space in the garden. Single rows of crops, while efficient on farms with large machines for planting, cultivating, and harvesting, are not always the best option in the backyard vegetable garden. The fewer rows you have in a home-sized garden, the fewer paths between rows you'll need, and the more square footage you'll have available to grow crops.

If your existing row garden is already producing enough food for you, switching to raised beds or open beds will allow you to downsize it. You can plant green-manure crops on the part of the garden that isn't currently growing vegetables, and/or rotate growing areas more easily from year to year, if you free up this existing garden space. Or, in the newly available space, you may discover that you have enough room to plant new crops such as rhubarb, asparagus, berries, or cutting flowers.

There are a number of other reasons to switch from rows to a dense garden.

one

system s ystem s ystem s system s ys

Effort is saved. Vegetables that are densely planted shade and cool the ground beneath them, requiring less watering, weeding, and mulching - in other words, less drudgery for the gardener.

Compaction of the soil is less. The more space between rows or beds you have, the more soil you and others will compact by walking through them. You will have more growing area that you won't be walking on if you increase the width of the growing beds and decrease the number of paths. This untrammeled soil will be fluffier and better for plant roots.

Grow up and don't be a slacker.

Trellising is the most efficient way to use space in the garden, aside from intensive planting. People with small gardens will want to grow as many crops as possible on vertical supports, while gardeners with plenty of space will still need to give some of their vegetables physical support, such as climbing peas and pole beans. Vining crops like cucumbers and tomatoes are commonly trellised as well.

So long as the crops grown on the fence can be rotated in different years, the fence surrounding your garden could serve as a trellis as well. Vegetable supplements come in a variety of forms.

12

Wood or metal are used to construct this piece. Regardless of the design or materials you choose, make sure your trellis is up and running well before the plants require it - preferably even before you begin planting the crop. Some plants, such as tomatoes or melons, may need to be gently tied to the support or weaved through the trellis as they grow.

Maintain Movement of Crops

Within the vegetable garden, crop rotation means only planting the same crop once every three years in the same spot. This policy ensures that the same garden vegetables don't deplete the same nutrients from year to year. It can also aid in the eradication of any insect pests or disease pathogens that may be lurking in the soil after the crop has been harvested.

Make a pian of the garden on paper during each growing season, showing the location of ali crops, if you're using a three-year crop rotation system. If you grow a lot of different vegetables, like most people, these garden plans will come in handy, because it can be difficult to remember what you were growing where even last season, let alone two years ago. You don't have to rely solely on memory because you've saved garden plans for the past two or three years.

A Constant Cropping

Another way to maximize growing space in the garden is to plan crops in succession. Gardeners all too often prepare their seedbeds and plant or transplant their crops in the spring on only one or two days, usually after the last frost date for their region.

While there's nothing wrong with planting a garden this way, wouldn't it be easier to plant a few seeds or transplants at a time over the course of the growing season, rather than taking on the herculean task of "getting in the garden" all at once?

Following Ali, the more you divide a job, the easier it becomes. From the first cold-hardy greens and peas in late winter or early spring to heat-loving transplants like tomatoes, peppers, and eggplant once the weather warms up and settles, Pian to plant something new in the garden almost every week of the season.

Then, depending on your climate, repeat the process by sowing frost-hardy y crops from mid-summer to mid-fall. As you harvest crops, continue to clean out the beds to make room for new vegetables to take their place. You can even sow the seeds of fast-growing crops like radishes alongside slower-growing vegetables like carrots and parsnips. Because you'll have already harvested the fast-growing crop and given the long-season 14 crop, thinning out the bed will be easier later on.

vegetables that still have a lot of room to move around in

Of course, succession planting has the added benefit of extending the harvest season for each crop. This means that, rather than being buried in snap beans or summer squash as your plants mature all at once, you can stagger your plantings to ensure a steady, but more manageable supply of fresh vegetables.

Maintain accurate records

Finally, we arrive at our starting point, with the realization that, while vegetable gardening can be rewarding even for novices, there is an art to doing it well. You can also find a wealth of useful information and advice from other gardeners. Paying close attention to how plants grow and keeping track of your successes and failures in a garden notebook or journal is one of the most important ways to improve your garden year after year.

Taking notes can help you avoid making the same mistakes again, or ensure that your good results can be replicated in future years, just like drawing a garden pian each year can help you remember where things were growing. For example, keep track of the narnes of various vegetable varieties and compare them year to year to see which ones clone best in your garden.

Many people keep a book in their car to keep track of their 15-year milestones.

routine maintenance, such as changing their oil. Similarly, make it a habit to write it down whenever you apply organic matter or fertilizer to your garden, or when you plant or begin harvesting a crop.

This type of careful observation and record-keeping will most likely teach you more about growing vegetables over time than any single book or authority. Because your notes will be based on your own personal experience and observations, they will reflect what works best for you in the unique conditions of your own garden. In the art of vegetable gardening, as in so many other endeavors, practice makes perfect.

16

Tomatoes

Tornatoes are easy to grow, prolific, versatile in the kitchen, and delicious straight from the vine. Choosing tornato varieties, starting seeds, transplanting tornatoes outside, using tornato stakes and cages, and tornato plant care are all covered in our guide.

Tornatoes are suo-lovers who grow slowly and seek heat. Frost does not affect these warren-seasoned plants. The soil is not warm enough in most areas until April or May, but this varies depending on where you live.

WHAT IS THE TIME IT TAKES FOR A TOMATO TO GROW?

17

One of our most frequently asked questions is about this. Days to maturity range from 60 to more than 80 days, depending on the cultivar.

Tomatoes are most commonly transplanted rather than seeded into the garden because they have a relatively long growing season. In garden nurseries, you can buy transplants. Short, stocky plants with dark green color and straight, sturdy stems the size of a pencil or thicker should be your target. Plants with yellowing leaves, spots, or stress damage should be avoided, as should those with flowers or fruits that are already ripening.

TOMATO CLASSIFICATION

Tomatoes come in a variety of sizes, ranging from tiny grape tomatoes to giant beefsteaks. The decision is also influenced by how you intend to prepare this versatile fruit. Roma tomatoes, for example, are not particularly tasty when eaten raw, but they work well in sauces and ketchups. The following are the different types of Tornato cultivars based on their growth habits:

• Determinate tomatoes are those that reach a specific height. They make excellent canning and sauce ingredients.

• Indicate tomatoes grow taller during the growing season because the stem termina l continues to grow.

instead of setting flower s, produce foliar growth These plants produce fruits all season long along the plant's side shoots. If you want to spread out your harvest over a longer period of time, indeterminate tomatoes are the way to go.

Because tomatoes are susceptible to pests and diseases, they require close attention. Select disease-resistant cultivars whenever possible to avoid problems. Also keep in mind that if you don't stake or support your tornato plants, they'll be more susceptible to soil-borne disease and rot. In the tornato guide below, we'll cover ali these essentials.

PLANTING

SEARCH FOR A SITE

Choose a sunny location. It is ESSENTIAL that your site receives at least 6 hours of daily sunlight in the northern hemisphere. Light afternoon shade will protect tomatoes from the harsh midday sun in southern climates, allowing them to thrive.

Tomatoes can grow in a variety of soils, but they must drain well and never collect water. A slightly acidic soil with a pH of 6.2 to 6.8 is ideal for them.

WHEN SHOULD TOMATOES BE PLANTED?

• Because tomatoes are not the easiest to start from seed, many gardeners start them from small plants or transplants purchased from a nursery.

• If you're growing tomatoes from seed, start them 6 to 8 weeks earlier than the average last spring frost date. For more information, see our Planting Calendar for specific seed-starting dates in your area, as well as our article "How to Grow Tomatoes From Seed."

• After the last spring frost has passed and the soil has warmed, transplant seedlings. For recommended transplanting dates, see our Planting Calendar.

TRAN SPLAN TIN G PRIOR TO TRAN SPLAN TRAN SPLAN TRAN SPLAN TRAN SPLAN

• Dig a 1 foot deep hole in the soil and mix in aged manure or compost two weeks before planting your tornato plants outside. More information on soil preparation for planting can be found here.

• Before planting seedlings or transplants in the garden, harden them off for a week. Set young plants outside for a couple of hours in the shade the first day, gradually increasing the amount of time they spend outside each day to include some direct sunlight.

• Place tornat o stakes o r cages in the soil at the time of planting to prevent root damage later. 20 are kept in stakes.

dev eloping tornato fruit off the ground, with caging allowing the plant to stand on its own. Use a strong pole with a diameter of 1 inch and a length of at least 8 feet for stakes. Place the pole about 4 inches away from the plant and 1 to 2 feet deep.

THE TRANSPLANT PLANTATION

• For every 100 square feet of garden area, apply 2 to 3 pounds of a complete fertilizer like 5-10-5, 10- 10-10, or 6-10-4. Applying high-nitrogen fertilizers, such as those recommended for lawns, is not recommended.

• Too much nitrogen promotes lush foliage but delays flowering and fruiting.

• For smaller bush-type plants or larger plants that will be staked, space tornato transplants 2 feet apart. If your plants aren't staked, space them out 3 to 4 feet apart. Allow for a distance of four feet between rows.

• On transplants, pinch off a few lower branches and plant the root bai! deep enough so that the remaining lowest leaves are just above the soil's surface.

•

If your transplants are leggy, bury up to 12 percent of the plant, including the lower leaves. The buried stems of tornato stems can produce roo ts.

• Make sure the transplant is well watered in order for it to thrive.

21

• Shade newly planted transplants for the first week or so to keep the leaves from drying out too much.

CONTAINER-GROWING TOMATOES

• Use loose, well-draining soil and a large pot or container with drainage holes in the bottom. A good potting mix with organic matter is recommended.

• In each pot, plant one tornato. Choose between bush and dwarf varieties; many cherry tomatoes thrive in containers.

• You may need to stake taller varieties.

• Place the pot in direct sunlight for 6 to 8 hours each day.

• Maintain a constant moisture level in the soil. Containers dry out faster than garden soil, so keep an eye on them daily and give them extra water during a heat wave.

CARE

HOW TO CARE FOR YOUR TOMATO PLANT

Watering

• Water well throughout the growing season, about 2 inches per 22 days, especially the first few days after the tornato seedlings or transplants are planted.

throughout the summer For a strong root system, water thoroughly.

• In the morning, drink some water. This provides the moisture that the plant requires to survive on a hot day. Late afternoon or evening, a void watering

• Mulch five weeks after transplanting to keep the soil moist and weeds at bay. Mulch also protects the lower tornato leaves from soil splashing. After the soil has had a chance to warm up, apply 2 to 4 inch es of organic mulch, such as straw, hay, or bark chips.

• Find some flat rocks and place one next to each plant to help tomatoes get through periods of drought. Water is stored in the rocks as a result of evapotranspiration from the soil.

Fertilizing

• Using a starter fertilizer solution to water in will help the roots get a head start.

• Fertilizer or compost should be applied every two weeks, beginning when the tornato fruits are about 1 inch in diameter.

• A nitrogen fertilizer sidedressing will aid in the visibility of the plants during the growing season. At each of the following times, apply one pound of ammonium nitrate (33-0-0) per 100 foot row:

23

• 1 to 2 weeks after first fruits are set • 2 weeks after picking first ripe fruit, and • 6 weeks after picking first ripe fruit.

•

If staking, use soft string or old nylon stocking to secure the tornato stem to the stake. It's essential to remove the suckers (side stems) by pinching them off just beyond the first two leaves. • If supporting tomatoes with a wire cage, suckers do not need to be removed. (This allows the plant to be more productive.)

• Practice crop rotation from year to year to prevent diseases that may have overwintered.

Weeding

• Where no mulch is used, cultivate shallowly to remove weeds while they are stili small. Herbicides can be used in large tornat o plantings but are not practical in the small garden with only a few plants of many different crops.

PESTS/DISEASES

Tornatoes are suscep tible to insect pests, especially tornato hornworrns and whiteflies. Click on links below to go to respective pest pages.

• Aphids

• Flea Beetles

• Tornato Hornworrn • Whiteflies • Blossorn-End Rot • Late Blight is a fungal disease that can strike during any part of the growing season. It will cause grey, rnoldy spots on leaves and fruit which later turn brown. The disease is spread and 25

support ed by persiste nt damp weather. Trus disease will ove rwinter, so all infected plants should be destro yed. See our blog on "Avo id Blight \X/ith th e Right Tornato ."

• Mosaic Virus creates disto rted leaves and causes young growth to be narrow and twisted, and the leaves become mottled with yellow. Unfor tunately, infected plants should be destro yed (but don't put them in your compost pile).

• Cracking: \X/hen fruir grow th is too rapid, the skin will crack. Trus usually occur s due to uneven watering or uneven moisture from weather condition s (very rainy periods mixed with dry period s). Keep moisture levels constant with co nsistent watering and mulcrung.

HARVEST/ STORAGE

HOW TO HARVEST TO MATOES

Leave yo ur tomatoes on the vine as long as possible. If any fall off before they appear ripe, piace them in a paper bag with the stem up and store them in a cool, dark piace.

Never piace tom atoes on a sunn y windowsill to ripen; they may rot before they are rip e!

The perfect tornato for picking will be firm and very red in color, regardless of size, with perhaps some yellow remaining around the 26

stern. If you grow orange, yellow or any other color tornato, wait for the tornato to turn the correct color.

If your tornato plant stili has fruit when the first hard frost threatens, pull up the entire plant and hang it upside down in the basernent or garage. Pick tornatoes as they ripen.

If temperatures start to drop and yo ur tomatoes aren't ripening, watch this video for tips.

You can harvest seeds from some tornato varieties. Learn how here.

HOW TO STORE TOMATOES

Never refrigerate fresh tomatoes. Doing so spoils the flavor and texture that make up that garden tornato taste.

To freeze, core fresh unblemished tornatoes and piace them whole in freezer bags or containers. Seal, label, and freeze. T he skins will slip off when they defrost.

RECOMMENDED VARIET IES

Tomat oes grow in many sizes, from tiny "cu rrant" to "cherry" to large " beefsteak." What's rnost irnportant is to look for disease- resistant cultivars whenever possible. Many modem cultivars have resistance to Verticillium wilt, Fusari um wilt, and root knot nernatod es. Cultivars with such resista nce are denoted as such by the 27

letters V, F, and following the cultivar name Here are a few of our favorite varieties of tomatoes: Early Varieties (60 or fewer days to harvest)

Early-maturing cultivars such as Early Girl may be slightly less flavorful but will produce fruit 2 to 3 weeks earlier than midor late- season cultivars.

'E arly Cascade': trailing plant, large fruit clusters

'E arly Giri': one of the earliest tomatoes, produces through the summer Mid-season

Varieties (70 to 80 days to harvest)

• 'Floramerica:' firm, deep red flesh, strong plant

• 'Fantastic': meaty rich flavor, heavy yields, crack resistant

Late-season Varietie s (80 days or more to harvest)

• 'Amish Paste': Large paste tomatoes, good slicers, heavy yields

• 'Brandywine': A beefsteak with perfect acid-sweet combination, many var iant s are available

Cherry Tomatoes

• 'Matt's Wild Cherry': bright red tomatoes, foolproof in any climate, bears abundant fruit in high or low temps and in rain or drought • 'Sun Gold':

golden orange tomatoes, very sweet yet tart flavor, huge clusters

Large Tomatoes

• Beefste ak, Beefmaster, Ponderosa, and Oxheart are noted for their large fruit.

However, these larger fruiteci types often are more susceptible to diseases and skin

cracking.

29

Squash (Zucchini)

Squash, especially zucchini, are outrageously pro lific prod ucer s! Easy to grow, each plant will produce severa! squash a day during peak season! Here's how to sow, grow, and harvest squash.

Chances are that you'll end up with more zucchini harvest that you can handle. But that's OK! See our recipes below for ali the clifferent ways you can enjo y (or preserve) zucchini. Plus, zucchini is full of nutrients! You can't go wrong.. .unless you forget to harvest and end up with giant baseball bats! (More on how to harvest later.)

Squash are generally divid ed into two categories based on when they're harvested and how they're used:

30

• Summer squash are warm-season crops harvested in the summer before they reach full maturity. Because they're harvested early, their skin is edible and they have a relatively sho rt shelf ! ife. Summer squash varieties include zucchini, yellow squash (straightneck squash), and crookneck squash. T

• Winter squash are harvested in autumn after or just before they reac h full maturity. This leaves their skin inedibl e, but gives them a longer shelf ! ife (some varieties are capable of keeping through the winter- hence the name "winter squash"). Winter squash varieties include pump kins, butternut squash, spaghetti squash, and acoro squash.

Most summer squash now come in bush varieties, which take up less space, but winter squash are vining plants that need more space. Bush varieties will nee d to be thinned in early stages of development to about 8 to 12 inches apart.

Thanks to their regular bumper crops, you usually o nJy need one or two zucchini plants- and yo u may stili find yourself g1v10g zucchini away to neighbors or baking lo ts of zucchini bread!

Would you believe that pumpkins and zucchini come from the same species of plant? T hat's right- they're both cultivated varieties ("cultivars") of Cucurbita pepo. D espite the great diversity of squash, most commonly-grown cultivars belong to one of three species: Cucurbit a pepo, C. moschata, or C. maxima. Over generations and generations, these plants have been cultivated to produce fruit in ali kinds of shapes, colors, and flavors.

PLANTING

WHEN TO PLANT SQUASH

• Sow squash/ zucc hini directly outsid e at least a week after your last frost date. The soil needs to be warm (at least 60°F/16°C at a two-inch depth) . The Garden Planner will calculate your exact planting dates for squash based on yo ur locatio n.

• lf you wish to start seeds indoors, sow 2 to 4 weeks befo re your last spring frost in peat pots.

• Warm the soil with black plastic mulch once the soil has been prepared in early spr ing.

• Do not rush. Waiting to plant will avoid problems from squash vine borers and other pests and diseases co mmo n earlier in the season.

CHOOSING AND PREPARING A PLANTING SITE

32

• Pick a spot with full sun, shelter from wind for good pollinations, and weli-draining soil.

• Squash plants are heavy feeders. Add plenty o f garden compost or weli-ro tted manure to the soil before planting.

• When you plant their holes, scatter in some organic fertilizer as weli.

HOW TO PLANT SQUASH

• Plant seeds in the ground about 1-inch deep and drop in 2 seeds. Pop a clear jar or half a plastic bottle over the top or use a cold frame protection in cold climates. Leave unti! the seedlings are up, and then remove the jar, and remove ali but the strongest seedling. • Alternatively, plant as a "hill" of 3 or 4 seeds sown d ose together on a small mound; this is helpful in northern climates, as the soil is warmer off the ground. Allow 5 to 6 feet becween hills.

• lf you wish to get a head start: Sow under cover in a greenhouse a couple wee ks earlier. Fili small pots or seed trays with potting mix and sew one seed in each pot.

Prepare smali plants for life outdoors by " hardening off." Set the pots outside fo r a week or two for a short time and increase the length of time. Plant after no risk of frost.

33

• Plant squash at least 2 feet apart. (fhe Garden Planner will calculate spacing for you.)

• T horoughly water after planting.

•

Adding a layer on top of mulch or organic matter can help lock in soil moisture.

CARE

HOW TO GROW SQUASH

• Mulch around plants to protect shallow roots, discourage weeds, and retain moisture.

• When the first bloo ms appear (which will be male flowers), apply a small amount of fertilizer as a side dre ss application.

• If your weather is cool, damp, or you're not seeing pollinators, you can hand pollinate your squash blossoms.

• For ali types of squ ash, frequent and consistent watering is important for good fruit development. Water most diligently when fruits form and throughout their growth period.

• Water deeply once a week, applying at least one inch of water. Do not water shallowly; the soil needs to be moist 4 inches down. • After harvest begins, fertilize occasio nally for vigorous growth and lots of fruits.

34

• If your fruits are misshapen, they might not bave received enough water or fertilization.

PESTS/DISEASES

Powdery Mildew can be a 1ssue on the leaves later on 1n the season. Keeping plants well-watered and leaving plenty of space between them for good air flow should slow the spread of this disease. If your squash does get powdery mildew, don't worry about it; plants will usually cope.

There are few challenging insect pests. The best solution is to get ahead of them before they arrive. Click on the links below to learn more.

Squash vine borer Squash bug Cucumber beetle Aplùds

Blossom-E nd Rot is an occasionai issue. If the blossom ends of your squash turn black and rot, then your squash have blossom-end rot. Tlùs condition is caused by uneven soil moisture levels, often wide fluctua tion s between wet and dry soil. It can also be caused by calcium levels. To correct the problem, water deeply and apply a truck mulch over the soil surface to keep evapo ration at a minim um. Keep the soil evenly moist like a wrung out sponge, not wet and not completely dried out.

HARVEST /STORAGE

HAVESTING SUMMER SQUASH

Begin harvesting zucc lùni and squash when the fruits are quite small (about 6 to 8 inches) Smaller fruits are more tender and flavorful with a denser, nuttier flesh. Believe us, smaller fruits have a far superior taste. If you have ever had a negative exper ience with zucc lùni before, it's probably beca use they were left to become bruisers.

Please, please, pl ease check every day on ce zucchini gets going.

Plus, picking frequently can lead to a larger crop.

Most varieties average 60 days to matur,it) , and are ready as soon as a week after flowe

ring. (Check the seed packet for more exact informatio n.)

Cut your squash from the vine with a sharp knife rather than breaking them off. Leave at

least an inch of stem on the fruit.

Should you miss a picking or two, remove the overr ipe sq uash as soon as possible to

reduce demands on the plants for moisture and nutrients.

Summer squash is very suscep tible to frost and heat damage, so you do want to pick

them ali befo re the first fall frosts arrive.

Store unwashed in the refrigerator unti! yo u' re ready to use. Fr es h summ er squash can

be stored in the refrigerator for up to ten days.

HARVESTING WINTER SQUASH

Harvest winter squash when the rind is hard and deep in color, usually late Septem ber

through October.

Winter squash can be stored in a cool, dark place unti! needed. Many varie ties will last for most of the winter (except for acorn squash, which do not keep for more than a few weeks). If you have a 37

cool bedroom, stashing them under the bed works well. They like a temperature of about 50 to 65°F (10 to 18°C).

Pull up the vines and compost them after you' ve picked everything or after a frost has killed them. Then till the soil to stir up the insects a bit.

RECOMMENDED VARIETIES

Summer Squash

'Cashflow': cylindrical zucchini type

'Cocozella (di Napoli)': zucchini heirloom; dark green, slender 'G oldbar': yellow surnmer squash

'Horn of Plenty': yellow crookneck type 'Sunb urst': pattypan/ scallop type 'Tigress': zucchini type

Winter Squash

'Butterbush': butternut, winter 'Buttercup': long vines, round fruit 'Cream of the Crop'
(acorn hybrid, winter) 38

'D elicata' is a bushy variety that is resistant to powdery mildew.

'Honeynut' is a butternut hybrid that yields smaller, more flavorful fruits.

'Tuffy' is an acorn variety with five to six fruits per plant.

'Waltham Butternut' has a big, tan fruit that increases in flavor as it ages.

Peppers (bell)

Peppers are pest-resistant and come in a variety of colors, shapes, and sizes, with something for everyone: spicy, sweet, or scorching. We'll concentrate on cultivating sweet beli peppers on this page.

Beli peppers, unlike their spicy cousins, lack capsaicin, the chemical that gives hot peppers its pungency and heat.

PLANTING

WHEN SHOULD PEPPERS BE PLANTED?

8-10 weeks before your final spring frost date, start seeds inside. Because beli peppers have a lengthy growth season (60 to 90 days), it's preferable to start them inside.

40

PLANTING SITE SELECTION AND PREPARE

To produce the biggest and healthiest fruit, pepper plants want full light, so choose a location that isn't covered by trees or other garden plants.

The soil should be well-draining and organic matter-rich.

A soil condition that is midway between sandy and loamy will drain effectively and warm up soon.

The pH of the soil should be acidic, preferably between 5.5 and 6.5.

Introduce fertilizer or old compost to your garden soil a week before transplanting peppers into the garden.

Planting peppers in areas where other nightshade family members, such as tomatoes, potatoes, or eggplants, have recently been produced might expose peppers to illness.

PEPPER SOWING INSTRUCTIONS

Rather of beginning seeds in the garden, we propose starting them inside. Seed germination requires a soil temperature of at least 70°F, so keep them in a warm environment for the best and quickest results. If required, place a heat pad beneath the seed tray.

Plant seeds at a depth of 14 inches.

41

Planting Young Plants in the Garden T ransplanting Young Plants in the Garden

Plants should be hardened off for around 10 days before being transplanted outside.

Transplant seedlings outside whenever overnight temperatures reach at least 60°F (16°C), spreading them 18 to 24 inches apart.

If you put the transplants any deeper than they were before, the stems may become susceptible to rot.

The soil temperature should be at least 65 degrees Fahrenheit, since peppers will not survive transplanting at temperatures lower than that. By covering the soil with black plastic, northern gardeners can warm it up.

CARE

PEPPER GROWING INSTRUCTIONS

Although the soil should be well-drained, take careful to keep it wet by mulching or covering it with plastic.

Water peppers once or twice a week, but keep in mind that they are particularly heat sensitive. If you reside in a hot or arid region, you may need to water your plants every day.

Fertilize following the initial ripening of the fruit.

To prevent damaging the roots of the plants, weed gently around them.

42

Support plants with cages or stakes if required to prevent be nding. Try co ne-shaped wire tornato cages, which are commercially available. They're not the best choice for tomat oes, but they're perfect for peppers. Build your own garden supports if you choose.

HARVESTING AND STOCKING

HOW DO YOU HARDEN PEPPERS?

As soon as the peppers reach the correct size or color, harvest them.

The longer beli p e pp ers remain on the plant, the sweeter they get and the more vitamin C they contain.

For the least amount of harm, cut peppers clean off the plant with a sharp knife or scissors.

HOW DO YOU KEEP PEPPERS?

After harvesting, peppers may be stored in plastic bags for up to 10 days.

Beli peppers may be dried, and we suggest using a regular oven for this. Peppers should be washed, cored, and seeded. Using a half-inch strip cutter, cut the dough into half-inch strips. After steaming for approximately ten minutes, lay out on a baking sheet. Dry until brittle, stirring regularly and swapping tray positions in the oven at 140°F (or the lowest allowable temperature). Place the peppers in bags or containers after they have cooled.

containers for storing

RECOMMENDED OPTIONS

Look for peppers that develop quickly to their full color; fully grown peppers are the most nutritious—and also the tastiest!

'Lady Beli,' 'Gypsy,' 'Beli Boy,' 'Lipstick,' 'Lady Beli,' 'Gypsy,' 'Beli Boy,' 'Lipstick,' 'Lady Beli,' 'Gypsy,' 'Beli Boy, 'Milena' and 'Orange Sun' are two orange varieties.

'Go lden California Wonder,' says YeUow.

44

Cabbage

G PLANTIN

Cabbage is a strong feeder that depletes the soil of essential nutrients fast.

Mix add old manure and/or compost to the soil ahead of time. Roots that stand in wet split or decay, therefore the soil should be well-draining.

Sow 14 inch deep 6 to 8 weeks before the final spring frost if beginning seeds indoors. For recommended planting dates, see our Planting Calendar.

Harden off the seedlings for a week before transplanting them to the outdoors.

2 to 3 45 t ransplant little plants outside on a cloudy afternoon

weeks before the final day of spring frost

Depending on the size of the desired head, space seedlings 12 to 24 inches apart in rows. The smaller the cabbages, the closer you plant them.

clirect Plant seeds outside (or plant transplants) in mid- to late summer for an autumn harvest. If your location is exceptionally hot and dry, wait until late summer to plant. Make sure your young plants don't dry out in the heat of the summer sun!

CARE

GROWING CABBAGES

Thin seedlings to allow the appropriate space between them when they reach around 5 inch es tali. If desired, move the trimmed seedlings to a new location.

46

Mulch heavily around the area to keep moisture in the soil and control the temperature. The ideal soil temperature for growth is 60 to 65 degrees Fahrenheit. Young plants that have been exposed to temperatures below 45°F for an extended length of time may bolt or have loose heads.

Fertilize with a balanced (10-10-10) fertilizer two weeks after transplanting.

Add a nitrogen-rich fertilizer three weeks late; cabbage need nitrogen in its early stages.

To minimize an accumulation of soil-borne illnesses, rotate your cabbage crops.

PESTS/DISEASES

According to traditional legend, strewing elder leaves over your cabbage would keep the pests away.

• Aphids • Cabbage Loopers • Cabbage Root Maggots • Cabbage Root Maggots • Imported Cabbageworms • Clubroot • Cutworms • Flea Beetles 47

Slugs/Snails • Stinkbugs • Thrips • D o wny Mildew

HARVEST/STORAGE

CABBAGE HARVESTING INSTRUCTIONS

Harvest when the heads have reached the required size and firmness. Heads that have matured will sp lighted. For most green cabbage cultivars, this will take roughly 70 days. The majority of early cultivars will yield 1- to 3-pound heads.

To harvest, use a sharp knife to cut each cabbage head at the base. Remove any yellow leaves (retain loose green leaves for storage protection) and bring the head inside or into the shade as soon as possible. Pull up the piane (roots and ali) alternately and 48

Hang it in a damp basement with temps around freezing.

Cut the cabbage head from the plant, leaving the outer leaves and root in the garden, to gain two harvests. New heads will appear on the plant; pluck them off until only four or five tiny heads remain. When the fruit reaches the size of a tennis ball (ideal for salads!), harvest it.

To avoid illness, remove the whole stem and root system from the soil after harvesting. Only compost healthy plants; those with maggot infestation should be destroyed.

CABBAGE STORAGE TIPS

Cabbage may be kept in the fridge for up to two weeks if lightly wrapped in plastic. Before storing, make sure it's completely dry. Cabbage may be stored for up to three months under optimal root celiar conditions. See our root celiars page for more information.

To get the most out of your cabbage crop, use this time-tested method:

Harvest the whole cabbage plant in the autumn, including the stems, head, and roots, and enjoy the head as normal while preserving the roots in a root cellar for the winter.

Plant the roots outside as soon as the gro und has thawed 1n spnng.

49

Fresh sprouts will appear soon, and they may be eaten alone or added to soups, salads, or any other recipe.

Although these replanted cabbages will not yield full heads, they should go to seed by the end of the summer, giving cabbage seeds for the following year!

Note: In the middle to late winter, this may be cloned inside on a windowsill; keep the roots wet and sprouts should appear.

RECOMMENDATION FOR DED VARIETY IE S

Cabbages are available in a variety of sizes, shapes, and colors.

• Try 'Primo' or 'Stonehead' for an early harvest.

• 'Go lden Acre' and 'Q uick Start,' which mature quickly, produce 3-pound heads.

• For Savoy varieties, try 'Alcosa,' an early variation, or 'Wirosa,' a late variety that overwinters as-is in southern gardens but requires care in the north. It's a heritage variety with slightly pointed heads and 2- to 3-pound heads.

'Blue Vantage' and 'Cheers' are two disease-resistant cultivars.

-

Try red or Chinese cabbage if you're growing for the autumn crop. 'Integro' and 'Ruby Perfection' (reds) and 'Li Ren Choy' (greens) are two excellent kinds (baby bok choy).

50

Beans, green

Green beans are a must-have in every vegetable garden since they're simple to cultivate, even in small spaces, and they're highly productive! Here's how to plant, cultivate, and harvest both pole and bush green beans.

Ali green beans are fragile annuals that are also known as "string beans" or "snap beans." Green beans come in a variety of colors, including purple, red, yellow, and streaked variants.

HOW DO BUSH BEANS AND POLE BEANS DIFFER?

The fundamental distinction among the different varieties of green beans is their shape.

51

if they have a "bush" or "pole" growth style

Bush beans grow compactly (to about two feet tali) and don't require additional support from a trellis.

Climbing vines, pomegranates can reach a height of 10 to 15 feet. Pole beans, as a result, need to be staked or trellised.

Learn how to properly supplement bea ns by watching this video. Of course, both types have their advantages and disadvantages:

Bush beans are easier to grow and require less upkeep, but pole beans produce more beans and are disease resistant.

Bush beans take 50 to 55 days to mature, while pole beans take 55 to 65 days to mature.

Bush beans often come in a bunch at once, so plant them every two weeks or so. Pole beans require the growth of their vines to produce, and if harvested regularly, will produce for a month or two.

PLANTING

WHEN SHOULD BEANS BE SEEDED?

When soils have warmed to at least 48°F (9°C), seeds can be sown outdoors any time after the last spring frost date. Plants should not be planted in excess of 52.

Because cold, moist soil slows germination and can cause seeds to rot, it's best to start planting early.

• Tip: Warm the soil with black plastic or scaping fabric to get a head start on planting.

Green bean seedlings should not be started inside. They may not survive transplanting because of their weak roots.

PLANTING SITE SELECTION AND PREPARATION

Beans thrive in fertile, well-draining soil. Beans do not require additional nitrogen fertilizer because they fix it themselves. Poor soil, on the other hand, should still be amended in the fall before planting with aged manure or compost.

Beans prefer soil pH levels that are slightly acidic to neutral (6.0- 7.0).

Before planting pole beans, set up any necessary supports.

BEANS AND HOW TO GROW THEM

• In rows 18 inches apart, sow bush bean seeds 1 inch deep and 2 inches apart. In sandy soil, plant a little deeper (but not too deep).

• Before planting pole beans, construct trellises or tepees to protect the delicate roots. 1 inch deep and 3 inches apart, plant pole bean seeds.

53

• Make a tepee by tying three to four (or more) 7-foot bamboo poles or long, straight branch es together at the top and splaying the legs in a circle. Then, around each pole, plant 3 to 4 seeds. Train the vines to climb the poles as they emerge. Wrap string/wire around the poles halfway up, encircling the tepee, for added stability; this provides something for the vines to grab.

• Tip: If you enjoy pole beans, a "cattle panel," which is a portable section of wire fence that is 16 feet long and 5 feet tall, is an easy way to support them. You won't have to get into contorted positions to pick the beans because they will climb easily.

•

Sow bean seeds every 2 weeks for a harvest that will last all summer. If you won't be able to harvest because you'll be away, don't plant. Beans are impatient!

• Rotate your crops to prevent pests and diseases from accumulating.

CARE

GREEN BEANS GROWING GUIDE

Mulch the soil around the bean plants to keep it moist and well-drained. Mulch helps keep beans cool because their roots are shallow.

54

2 inches of water per week is recommended. Beans will stop flowering if they are not kept well watered. On hot days, water the foliage to prevent it from drying out and becoming disease-prone.

If necessary, begin fertilizing after heavy bloom and the set of p o d s. Avo id using high-nitrogen fertilizer or you will get lush foliage and few beans. A side dressing of co mpost or composted manure halfway th rough the growing season is a good alternative to liquid fertilizer.

Weed dilige ntly but carefully to preve nt disturbing the shallow root systems of the beans.

Pinch off the tops of pole bean vines when they reach the top of th e s upport. This will for ce them to put energy into producin g more pods instead.

In high heat, use row covers over young plants; hot weather can cause blo sso ms to drop from plants, reducing harvest.

PESTS/ DISEASES

Anthracnose Aphids\sCucum ber Beetles

Cutworms

Japanese Beetles

Mexican Bean Beetles (These beetles eat the flowers, beans and especially leaves of beans) (These beetles eat the flowers, beans and especially leaves of beans.)

Powdery Mildew

Mosaic Viruses (Try to keep vines dry by not crowding plants and providing ample air circulation) (Try to keep vines dry by not crowding plants and providing ample air circulation)

Slugs/Snail (These pests are attraeteci to damp conditions) (These pests are attraeteci to damp conditions.) White Mold (Avoid damp conditions) (Avoid damp conditions)

Whiteflies Woodchucks

HARVEST /STORAGE

HOW TO HARVEST GREEN BEANS

Harvest beans in the morning when their sugar level is highest.

Green beans are picked young and tender before the seeds inside have fully developed.

Pick green beans every day; the more you pick, the more beans grow.

56

Look for firm, sizable that are firm and can be snapped- generally as thick as a pencil.

Snap or cut the beans off the plant, being careful not to tear the plant. Fresh beans should snap easily when broken.

Once you see the seeds inside bulging, green beans are past their peak and will taste tough.

HOW TO STORE GREEN BEAN S

Stare beans in a moisture-proof, airtight container in the refrigerator. Beans will toughen aver time even when stored properly.

Beans can be kept fresh for about 4 days, or blanched and frozen irnmediately after harvesting.

Beans can also be canned or pickled.

RECOMMEN DE D VARIETIES

When it comes to green beans, the options are endless. Here are some types and varieties to consider:

• Chinese (aka Asian) long beans (aka yardlong or asparagus beans): slender 1- to 2-foot pods. Try 'O rient Wonder', 'Red Noodle', or 'Yardlong.' Ali pale.

• French green beans (aka filet or haricot verts): thin, tender,

57

3- to 5-inch pods. Try 'Calima', 'Masai', or 'Maxibel'; in a container, plant 'Mascotte'. Ali bush.

• Italian / Romano: wide, flat 6- to 8-inch pods even in the hottest summers. Try 'Early Bush Italian ', extra- large-pod 'Jum bo', or 'Roma II'. Ali bush.

• Purple beans: 5- to 6-inch pods are deep purpose when raw and turn green when cooked. Tr y 'Amethyst', 'Royal Burga ndy', or 'V elour'. Ali bush.

• Snap beans (aka string or stringless): slender, 5- to 7-inch pods. Try 'Blue Lake 274' (bush), heirloo m 'Ken tucky Wonder' (bush or pole), or 'Provider' (bush) (bush).

• Yellow wax beans: 5- to 7-inch pods with a milder flavor than green varieties. Try stringless 'C herokee' (bush), classic 'G olden Wax' (bush), or 'Monte Gusto' (pole) (pole).

Lettuce

Lettuce is one of our favorite garden vegetables because it is far superi o r- in both taste and vitam in A content-to thestore-bought alternative! Plant in the spring, starting two weeks before frost. In fall, start sowing again eight wee ks before the fall frost.

Lettuce is cool-season crop that grows well in the spring and fall in mo st regions. Lettuce seedlings will even tolerate a light frost.

Sow any time soils are above 40°F. Seeds germinate best at 55 to 65°F and will emerge in only 7 to 10 days. Because lettuc e grows quickly, plant a small amount at a time, staggering your plantings to a continued harvest!

59

PLANTING

HOW TO PLANT LETTUCE

Before you plant your lettuce seeds, select a sunny spot and make sure the soiJ is prepared.

The soil should be loose and drain well so it's moist without staying soggy. To keep the soil fertile, feed it with composted organic matter about one week before you seed or transplant. Since the seed is so small, a well-tilled seedbed is essential. Stones and large clods of dirt will inhibit germination. Read more about preparing soil for planting.

Lettuce does not compete well with weeds. Before you piane, ensure the ground is prepared. Rotating locations from year to year\s60

helps contro! most diseases. Closely spaced plants will help contro! weeds.

Direct sowing is recommended as soon as the ground can be worked. If you want an earlier crop, however, you may start seeds indoors 4 to 6 weeks before your last spring frost date for an earlier crop .

Lettuce can be sown after soils reach 40°F though seeds germinate best at 55 to 65°F and will emerge in 7 to 10 days.

Seeds should be planted ¼-½ inch deep and thinned when plants have 3 to 4 true leaves.

Transplants should have 4 to 6 mature leaves and a well-developed root system before planting out.

Transplants should be planted near the last frost-free date for the growing area. Seeded lettuce may be planted 2 to 3 weeks earlier.

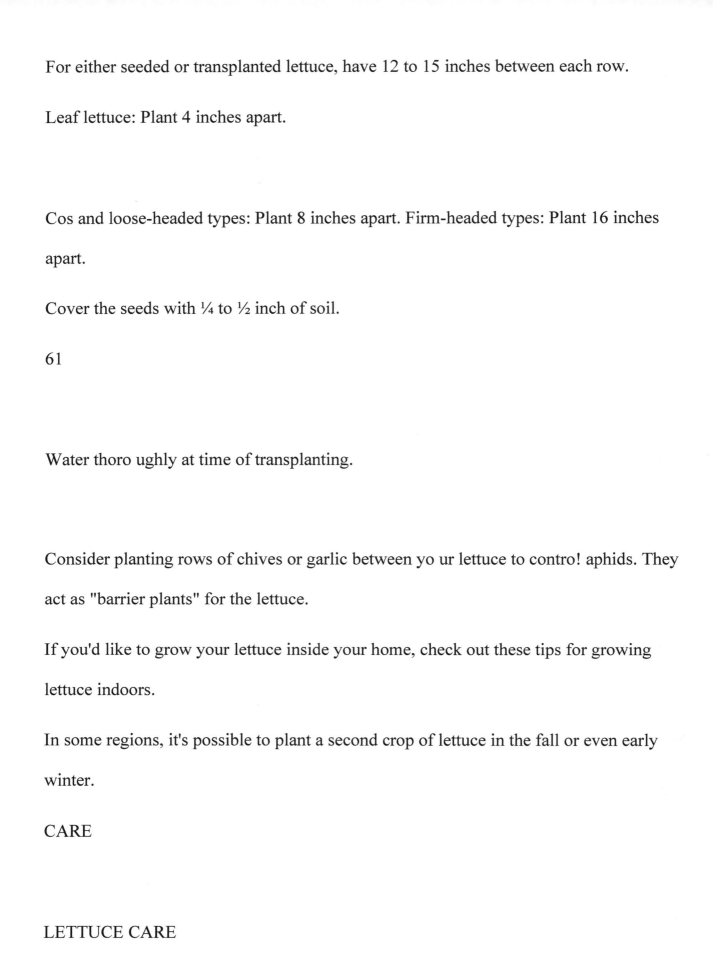

For either seeded or transplanted lettuce, have 12 to 15 inches between each row.

Leaf lettuce: Plant 4 inches apart.

Cos and loose-headed types: Plant 8 inches apart. Firm-headed types: Plant 16 inches apart.

Cover the seeds with ¼ to ½ inch of soil.

61

Water thoro ughly at time of transplanting.

Consider planting rows of chives or garlic between yo ur lettuce to contro! aphids. They act as "barrier plants" for the lettuce.

If you'd like to grow your lettuce inside your home, check out these tips for growing lettuce indoors.

In some regions, it's possible to plant a second crop of lettuce in the fall or even early winter.

CARE

LETTUCE CARE

Fertilize 3 weeks after transplanting. Lettuce prefers soil that is high in organic material, with plenty of compo st and a steady supply of nitrogen to keep if growing fast. Use organic alfalfa meal or a slow-release fertilizer.

Make sure the soil remains moist but is well drained.

Lettuce will teli you when it needs water. Just look at it. If the leaves are wilting, sprinkle them anytime-even in the heat of the day- to cool them off and slow down the transpiration rate.

An organic mulch will help conserve moisture, suppress weeds, and keep soil temperatures cool througho ut the warmer months.

62

Weed by hand if necessary, but be careful of damaging yo ur lettuce plants' roots; they are shallow.

Planning your garden so that lettuce will be in the shade of taller plants, such as tomatoes or sweet com, may reduce bolting in the heat of the summer.

You should be able to sow additional lettuce seeds every two weeks for a continuous harvest throughout the growing season.

To plant a fall crop, create cool soil in August by moistening the ground and covering it with a bale of straw. A week later, the soil under the bale will be about 10°F (6°C) cooler than the rest of the garden. Sow a three-foot row of lettuce seeds every couple of weeks-just rotate the straw bale around the garden.

PESTS/DISEASES

• Aphids\s• Earwigs\s• Cutworms\s• White Mold\s• Woodchucks\s• Rabbits

HARVEST /STORAGE

63

HOW TO HARVEST LETTUCE

Lettuce should be harvested when full size, but just before maturity. The leaves taste best when they're stili yo ung and tender.

Before maturity, you can harvest leaf lettuce by simply removing outer leavesso that the center leaves can continue to grow.

Butterhead or romaine types can be harvested by removing the outer leaves, digging up the whole plant, or cutting the plant about an inch above the soil surface. A second harvest is often possible when using the first or third methods.

Crisphead lettuce is picked when the center is firm.

Mature lettuce gets bitter and woody and will go bad guickly, so check your ga rden everyday for read y-to- harvest leaves.

l t's best to harvest lettuce in the morning before leaves have been exposed to sun.

As time passes and the plant loses vigor, you may be better off planting a second round of seeds than waiting for new leaves.

Keep lettuce in the refrigerator for up to 10 days in a loo se plastic bag.

VARIETIES RECOMMENDED

• Some of our favorite varieties include:

• Crisphead: 'King Crown', 'Mission'

• Cos (Romaine): 'Wallop', 'Paris White Cos'

• Loose Heads: 'Burpee Bibb'

• Red Leaf: 'Red Sail' (Not recommended for hot weather; the red pigment absorbs more heat.)

And there are so many more types of lettuce to explore!

65

Beets

A staple in our garden, beets grow easily and yo u won't have to wait long until harvesting their tasty roots. And yo u can eat their green tops, too, so they're a dual-purpose crop. Learn ali yo u need to know about growing beets- from planting to harvest!

Beets or " beet roots" are a colorful, cool-season crop that is easy to grow from seed in well-prepared soil- and grows quickly in bright sun.

They are a great choice for northern gardeners because they can survive frost and near-freezing tempe ratures.

If you are a beginner, look for bolt-resistant varieties, which have less of a chance of bolting (ma turing too quickly) in warm weather.

66

T here are many di fferent varieties of beets, showcasing deep red, yellow, white, or striped roots of different shapes.

Beet roots can be harvested fro m the time they' re abo ut the size of a golf ball to the size of a tennis ball; larger roo ts may be tough and woody. Plu s, beet gree ns have a delicious and distinctive flavor and hold even more nutrition than the roo ts!

PLANTING

WHEN TO PLANT BEETS

Start your first round of beets in early spring, as soon as the soil is workable. Make successive plantings every 2 to 3 weeks until mid- summer.

Success ive plantings are possible as long as daytime temperatures don't exceed 75°F.

In soil that's at least 50°F (10°C), germination takes piace in 5 to 8 days. In soil colder than 50°F, germination may take 2 to 3 weeks.

• Tip: To speed up germinatio n, or when plan ting in areas with low moisture and rainfall, soak the seeds in water for 24 hours before planting.

Winter crops are a definite possibility in Zo ne 9 and warmer. Plant beets in early to late fall for a winter harvest.

67

PLANTING SITE SELECTION AND PREPARATION

Plant beets in full sun.

Beets prefer well-prepared, fertile soil but will also tolerate average to low soil fertility.

To allow beet roots to develop properly, so il sho uld be free of roc ks and other obstacles.

Soil pH between 6.0 and 7.0 is best and slightly alkaline (7.0+) soils can be tolerated. Beets do not tolerate soil with a low pH (below 6.0). (below 6.0).

If you fertilize, go easy o n nitrogen; excess will cause an abundance of greens but tiny bulbs beneath the soil. Learn more about soil amendments and preparing soil for planting.

HOW TO PLANT BEETS\s68

We prefer to sow beets clirectl y in the garden so that we don't have to disturb their roots, though beets- unlike many root crops- do generally tolerate being transplanted while stili yo ung. However, since they are cold tolerant, beets typically have no trouble being started outdoors.

Sow seeds ½-inch deep and 1 to 2 inches apart in rows that are about 1 foot apart. After sowing, cover the seeds with a thin layer of soil.

Each wrinkled beet "seed" is actualiy a cluster of 2 to 4 seed s, so you will need to thin the young plants to 3 to 4 inches apart once the greens get to be about 4 inches tali.

Tip: When thinning, don't pull up the plants, as you may accidentally clist urb the roots of the beets you want to kee p. In stea d, just snip off the greens (and eat them) (and eat them).

Make sure soil remains moist for optimal germination. Soak seeds for 24 hours prior to planting to speed up germination.

CARE

HOW TO GROW BEETS

Thinning is necessary, as you may ge t more than one seedling out of each seed. When the tops are a 4 to 5 inches tali, thin seedlings to\s69

3 to 4 inches apart. Pinch or cut off the leaves. Pulling them out of the groun d may disturb the roots of nearby seedlings .

Mulch and then water regularly with about 1 inch per week. Beets need to maintain plenty of moisture.

Weed as needed but be gentle; beets have shallow roots that are easily disturbed.

PESTS/ DISEASES

HARVEST/STORAGE • Flea Beetles • Leaf Miners • Leaf Spot • Cercospora • Leafhoppers • Mosaic Virus

BEES HARVESTING INSTRUCTIONS

The majority of types have a maturity period of 55 to 70 days.

To put it another way, beets should be harvested roughly two months after they are planted.

When roots are the size of a golf ball or greater, they are ready to harvest; particularly large roots might be stiff and woody.

Pull the beet out of the ground by loosening the dirt surrounding it.

70

Beet greens may be harvested at practically any time, although it's best to start when seedlings are thinned. Take one or two mature leaves per plant until the leaf blades have grown to a length of more than 6 inches and have become tough. (Roots cannot completely grow without greens, thus some should be left to ensure appropriate development.)

Red and white beet rings

HOW TO KEEP BEETS SAFE IN THE STORAGE ROOM

Beets may be preserved for 5 to 7 days in the refrigerator.

Beets will stay fresher for longer if the tops are clipped off. Leave approximately an inch of stem on each beet and keep the greens apart from the beets.

Brush off any dirt sticking to the roots before burying them in layers (but not touching) and surrounded by dry sand or sawdust for long-term root celiar storage.

Keep cool and dry. Put them in a cold basement or an unheated closet. Learn more about a novel method for storing beets in the root cellar.

Sprouting is an indication of insufficient storage, which leads to deterioration. You can also freeze, can, and pickle beets.

DED VARIETIES SHOULD BE RECOMMENDED AGAIN

71

Beets are available in a wide variety of forms and hues. The most common color is deep red, although yellow and white variations, as well as red-white ringed versions (as shown above), are also available.

• 'Detroit Dark Red': A classic varietal with a strong foundation. Red root, round in shape.

• 'Formanova' beets are long, cylindrical beets that grow like carrots. Canning from a distance is fantastic.

• 'Chioggia': crimson skin with red and white concentric bands visible when cut open.

• Yellow variants include 'Bolder' and 'Touchstone Gold; white variations include 'Avalanche' and the Dutch heritage 'Albino.'

Carrots

The taste and texture of garden-grown carrots are incredible! They're a popular, long-lasting root vegetable that thrives in a variety of climes. Learn how to grow, harvest, and sow carrots with Ali.

Carrots are simple to grow if planted in loose, sandy soil throughout the colder months of the growing season, such as spring and autumn (carrots can tolerate frost). Carrots may take anywhere between 2 and 4 months to mature, depending on the type and growing circumstances.

GOOD SOIL IS VERY IMPORTANT.

For carrot cultivation, proper soil preparation is essential! Stunted and deformed harvests might result if the carrot roots cannot readily develop unhindered.

To prepare your garden soil, follow these instructions:

• Till down 12 inches and check for rocks, stones, or even dirt clumps that might stymie the development of your carrots.

• Work in old coffee grounds instead of nitrogen-rich materials like manure and fertilizer, which may lead carrots to fork and sprout little side roots.

• Carrots should be planted on a raised bed that is at least 12 inches deep and filled with fluffy, sandy, or loamy soil if the soil is heavy d ay or too rocky (not d ay nor silt).

• Finally, don't expect groce ry sto re carrots to be perfectly shaped. Regardless of their form, your carrots will taste great!

PLANTING

Directly sow seeds in pots or in the garden. Transplanting is not advised. Use a seed-sower or thin forcefully to the correct space if you want to scatter seed in an equal manner so seeds don't grow together.

Carrots like full sun, but may grow in moderate shade.

To allow carrot roots to readily push down into the earth, the soil must be loose, sandy, and airy, as previously stated.

3–5 weeks before the final spring frost date, sow seeds outside.

Here you can find out when the frosts are expected in your area.

Sow 14 inches deep in rows 1 foot apart, 3 to 4 inches apart.

To prevent the formation of a crust, cover with a layer of vermiculite or fine compost (which would hamper germination).

Sow seeds every three weeks to get multiple harvests.

Using frequent shallow waterings, keep the soil moist. The soil must not form a hard crust on top for small carrot seeds to germinate. (If you stick your finger in the ground until the middle knuckle, it should be moist but not wet.)

Carrots are notorious for taking a long time to sprout. It may take 2 to 3 weeks for them to sprout leaves, so don't get discouraged if your carrots don't sprout right away!

Mix carrot seeds with fast-germinating radish seeds or sow radish seeds in rows between carrot rows to aid in spotting the first appearance of their tiny leaves.

CARE

Mulch carrots lightly to help them retain moisture, germinate faster, and keep the sun off their roots.

Thin seedlings to 3 to 4 inches apart once they've reached an inch tali. To avoid damaging the remaining plants' fragile roots, snip the tops off with scissors rather than pulling them out.

\

To begin, xfater one inch per week, then two inches as the roots mature.

Carefully weed, taking care not to disturb the roots of the young carrots.

Fertilize 5 to 6 weeks after sowing with a fertilizer that is low in nitrogen but high in potassium and phosphate. (It's important to note that too much nitrogen in the soil encourages top growth, not root growth.)

More carrot-growing advice is available here.

PESTS/DISEASES

• Carrot rust flies • Flea Beetles • Root-knot nematodes • Wireworms • Black (Itersonilia) canker • Carrot rust flies • Flea Beetles

Shortened and discolored carro t tops, as well as hairy roots, are signs of Aster Yellow Disease. Pests carry the disease from plant to plant when they feed. Keep weeds at bay and invest in a pest-control strategy for leafhoppers, for example. This disease is capable of surviving the winter.

STORAGE AND HARVEST

The taste of carrots is generally better when they are smaller.

Harvest when the desired maturity/size is reached, which is at least 12 inches in diameter and the size of your finger.

If you're growing carrots in the spring or early summer, harvest them before the daily temperatures rise too high, as heat can cause carrots to become fibrous.

After one or a few frosts, carrots taste much better. (A frost encourages the plant to begin storing energy in the form of sugars in its roots for 77 days.)

) Cover carrot tops with an 18-inch layer of shredded leaves after the first hard frost in the fall to keep them alive for later harvesting.

Carrots are only available once every two years. If you don't harvest your carrots and leave them in the ground, the tops will flower the following year, producing seeds.

FRESH CARROTS: HOW DO YOU KEEP THEM?

To store freshly harvested carrots, twist or cut off all but 12 inch of the tops, scrub any dirt off with cold running water, and air-cry. Refrigerate the sealed airtight plastic bags. Fresh carrots will go limp in a matter of hours if simply placed in the refrigerator.

If the ground does not freeze and pests are not a problem, you can leave mature carrots in the soil for temporary storage.

78

Carrots can also be stored in cool, dry areas in tubs of moist sand or sawdust.

VARIETIES RECOMMENDED

• Carrots are available in a wide variety of colors, sizes, and shapes.

• "Bolero": slightly tapered; 7–8 inches; resistant to most leaf pests and blights

• 'Danvers': a classic heirloom with a rich, dark orange color and a 6 to 8 inch length that tapers at the end; suited to heavy soil.

• 'Little Finger': heirloom; a small Nantes carrot with a diameter of 4 inches and a thickness of 1 inch; excellent for containers.

• 'Na ntes': cylindrical (not tapered); 6 to 7 inches; extremely sweet; crisp texture

• 'Th umberline' is an heirloom round carrot that grows well in clumpy or dry soil and containers.

•

Try heirloom 'Red Cored Chantenay' and bright 'Solar Yellow' for an unusual color combination.

Chard de Suisse

The Swiss ch ard, also known as "ch ard," is a beet that thrives in both cool and warm climates. Here's how to grow Swiss chard in your own backyard!

The stems of Swiss chard come in a rainbow of colors, including pink, yellow, orange, red, and white. Even if you don't care for chard's flavor, it can be used as a lovely ornamental plant!

Chard is a quick and easy to grow vegetable that can be cooked or eaten raw. The plant is also high in vitamins A, C, and K, making it an excellent addition to any diet.

Leaf beet, seakale beet, silver beet, and spinach beet are some of the other names for chard.

PLANTING

WHEN SHOULD SWISS CARD BE PLANTED?

Because it grows best in the cooler temperatures of spring and fall, Swiss chard is typically grown as a cool-season crop. Chard, on the other hand, can tolerate a wider range of temperatures. Its growth will slow in the summer, but chard's higher heat tolerance makes it a great salad green to grow when the weather gets too hot for other salad greens.

2–3 weeks before the last spring frost date, sow chard seeds.

Chard is best grown as a cut-and-come crop. This method of harvesting involves only taking a few older leaves from each plant at a time, leaving younger leaves to continue growing for later harvests. Plant adjcio nal chard seeds at 10-day intervals for about a month in the spring if you prefer to harvest the entire plant at once.

Plant chard seeds 40 days before the first frost date in the fall for a fall harvest.

81

PLANTING SITE SELECTION AND PREPARATION

Chard grows best in full sun, but will tolerate partial shade.

By mixing m compost before planting, you can ensure that your soil is well-draining and rich. Use a balanced fertilizer (10-10-1O) on the planting site if your soil is particularly poor.

Chard grows best in soil with a pH of 6.0 to 7.0 (a little acidic to neutral!).

SWISS CHARD PLANTING GUIDE

Soak seeds in water for 24 hours before planting to speed up the germination process.

Seeds should be sown 12 to 1 inch deep and 2 to 6 inches apart in rows.

18 inches between rows is a good distance.

Chard seeds, like beet seeds, come in clusters of a few seeds, resulting in multiple seedlings emerging from a single planting hole.

Thin the plants to about 6 to 8 inches apart once they reach a tali of 3 to 4 inches (or 9 to 12 inches apart if yo u desire larger plants). Snip the seedlings with scissors and eat them as a snack!

adverbial adverbial adverbial Because chard is grown for its leaves, thinning isn't as critical as it is for beets, which need room to expand their large, round roots. Chard plants that are overcrowded tend to produce fewer leaves.

CARE

GROWING SWISS CHARD

Chard grows well without fertilizer, but if your plants are still small halfway through the season, apply a balanced fertilizer.

To aid in the growth of Swiss chard, water it evenly and consistently. During the summer, water your plants frequently. To help conserve moisture, mulch the plants.

Cut the plants back to about 1 foot tali for the best quality. The flavor of chard plants decreases as they grow larger.

PESTS/DISEASES

Slugs • Aphids • Leaf miners

STORAGE AND HARVEST

SWISS CHARD HARVESTING GUIDE

Harvesting can begin when the plants reach a height of 6 to 8 inches, depending on the size of leaves desired. With a sharp knife, cut off the outer leaves 1 to 12 inches above the ground (avoiding damaging the plant's center).

Harvest the largest, oldest leaves and leave the younger ones to continue growing using the "cut-and-come-again" technique. New leaves will grow and provide another harvest if you harvest them carefully.

The ribs of chard leaves can be cut off and cooked in the same way as asparagus.

Greens are made from the remaining leaves. You can eat them raw or prepare them like spinach.

WHERE SHOULD SWISS CHARD BE KEEPED?

Swiss chard leaves should be rinsed and stored in ventilated plastic bags in the refrigerator.

VARIETIES RECOMMENDED

• 'Bright Lights': Dark green leaves on multicolored stems; resistant to bolting but frosty.

• 'Fo rdh ook Giant': compact plants with dark green leaves and white stems.

• 'Lucullus': Heat-tolerant plant with green leaves and white stems.

• 'Peppermint': Green leaves with pink and white striped stems; bolt resistant; container friendly.

• 'Rainbow' leaves and stems come in a rainbow of colors: red, pink, white, yellow, orange, and striped.

• 'Rhubarb': Dark green leaves with deep red stems; sow after the danger of frost has passed or it will bolt.

• 'Ruby Red': Green leaves with bright red stems; sow after the risk of frost has passed or the plant will bolt.

Radishes

Radishes are a hardy, low-maintenance root vegetable that can be planted several times during the growing season. Radishes can also be harvested as early as three weeks after they are planted! Our complete guide to growing radishes in your garden can be found here.

Radish seeds can be planted in the spring and fall, but growth should be halted during the summer months, when temperatures are typically too hot. (Radishes can bolt in hot weather, rendering them useless.)

Radishes, on the other hand, are one of the simplest vegetables to cultivate.

PLANTING

CHOOSING AND READYING A PLANTATION SITE

Place your plant in the sun. Radishes will put all of their energy into producing larger leaves if they are planted in too much shade, or even where neighboring vegetable plants shade them.

Radish plants are grown primarily for their roots, similar to carrots. The soil should be rich in organic matter but not compacted. If your soil is clay-like, add some sand to loosen it up and improve drainage.

If your soil is lacking in organic matter, add a few inches of aged compost or all-purpose fertilizer to the planting site as soon as it is workable (see packaging for amount).

87

Before you start planting, till your garden bed to get rid of any rocks or clods.

Rotate your crops every three years. To put it another way, radishes should only be planted every third year in the same location. This will aid in the prevention of disease in your crop.

RADISH PLANTATION INSTRUCTIONS

Sow seeds 4-6 weeks before the average last frost date in the spring for a spring planting. Find out when the locai frosts.

To avoid disturbing the roots of radish plants, plant the seeds directly in the garden. Sow seeds directly outside in rows 12 inches apart, 12 to 1 inch deep and 1 inch apart.

Plant a new round of seeds every 10 days or so, while the weather is still cool, to ensure a steady supply of radishes in the late spring and early summer.

Pianist Pianist Pianist Pianist Pianistic Pianistic Pianistic Pian Radishes can be planted later in the summer or early fall than any other root crop and still produce a harvest. Seeds should be planted 4-6 weeks before the first frost of the fall season.

CARE

RADISH GROWING GUIDE

When the plants are a week old, thin radishes to about 2 inches apart. Plants that are crowded don't thrive.

Moisture that is constant and even is critical. Maintain an even moisture level in the soil while avoiding over-watering. Drip irrigation is a fantastic way to accomplish this.

In dry conditions, a thin layer of mulch applied around the radishes can help retain moisture.

PESTS/DISEASES

Weeds: Weeds will quickly crowd out radishes, so keep the bed free of them. Here's a list of some of the most common weeds in the garden.

STORAGE AND HARVEST

RADISH HARVESTING INSTRUCTIONS AND EXAMPLES

Radishes mature quickly, with some varieties ready to harvest as soon as three weeks after planting.

Harvest when the roots are about 1 inch in diameter at the soil surface for the majority of varieties. Before harvesting the rest, pull one out and test it!

Radishes should not be left in the ground after they have reached maturity;

Their condition will quickly degrade.

Remove the tops and thin root tails, then wash and thoroughly dry the radishes. In the fridge, they're stored in plastic bags.

Separately stored radish greens can last up to three days.

VARIETIES RECOMMENDED

'French Breakfast' is a late-maturing variety that handles moderate heat well.

'Watermelon' is a sweet, mild radish with a pinkish center and white skin.

'Burpee White' has a white skin and is a spring variety.

'D aikon' is a white Japanese "winter radish" that can grow to be quite large (up to 2 feet in diameter).

(16 in.). In cooler climates or at the end of the growing season, this variety performs best.

'Rat's Tail' radishes are grown for their seedpods, not their roots. The pods have a stronger tangy, spicy flavor than regular radish.

'Dragon's Tail' radishes are grown for their seedpods, just like 'Rat's Tail'. This variety's pods are thinner and turn a beautiful purple color as they mature.

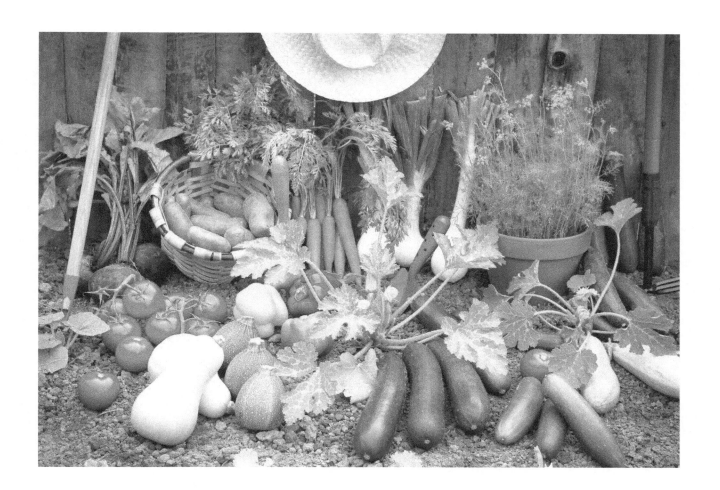

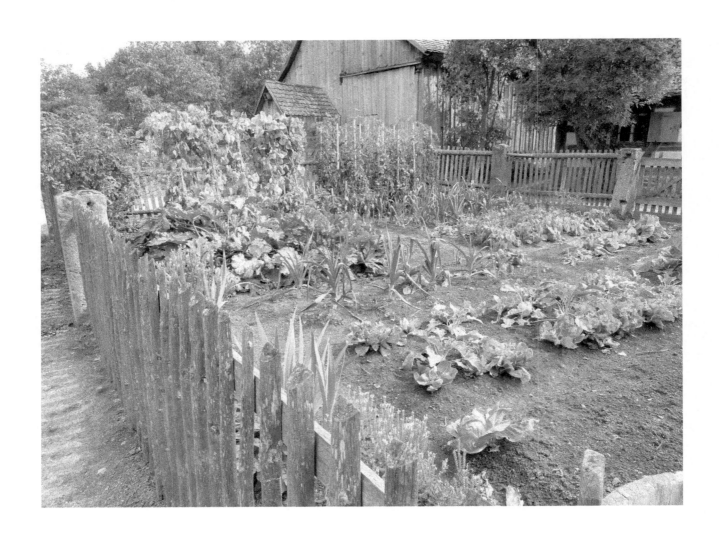

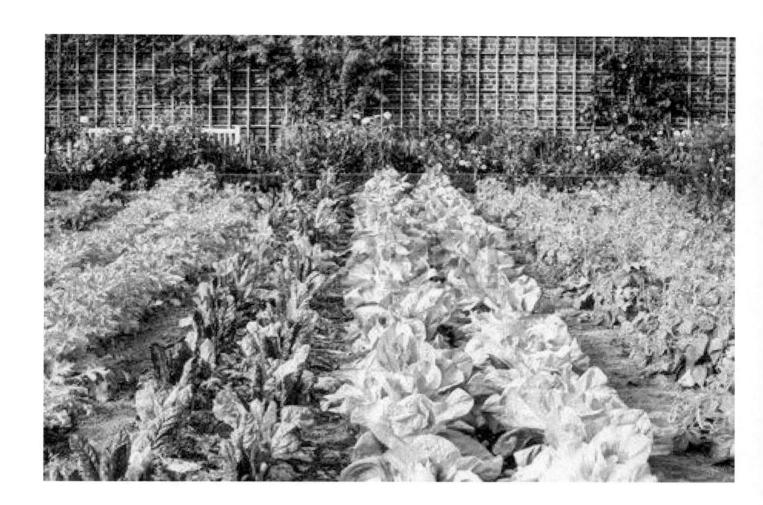

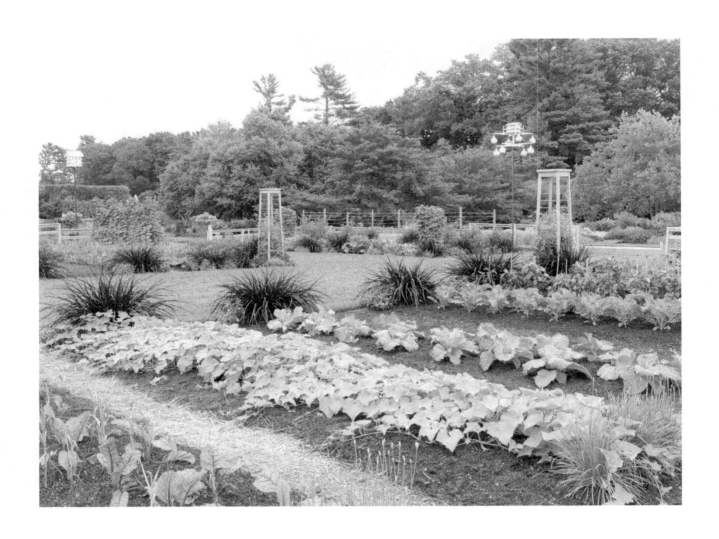

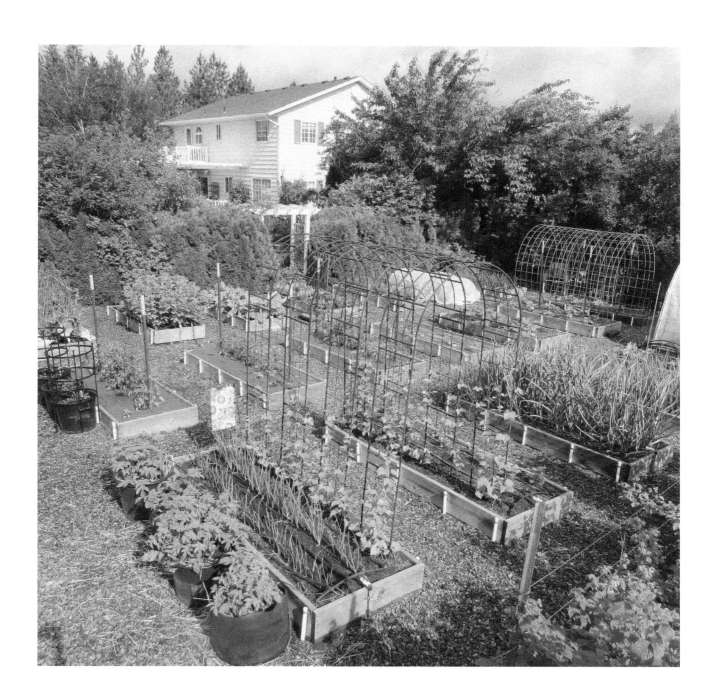

CPSIA information can be obtained
at www.ICGtesting.com
Printed in the USA
BVHW011105170222
629335BV00007B/204